BURNT!

By

Lori Osterloh Hagaman

Special thanks to my family for putting up with me while engaged in this book. An extra special thanks to my friend Jasmine for aiding in editing and lending a nurse's input.

I had this book almost finished. Then my onlaptop caught on fire. Yes, it literally caught on fire. After my husband, the techy guru of the two of us, pronounced the charred remains impossible to resurrect, and my two week period of mourning was over, I came to the realization that the Higher Power wanted me to revamp my work. I really had slap-dashed through the project. The tone was a bit snarky and a lot of it was choppy or hard to follow.

So here is a work that is reborn from the fire just as the mythical Phoenix. Let's hope this time I get it right, so as to not crash and burn again. I made myself chuckle there. Hopefully you got a slight rise out of that, too. That is what this work is all about. The "burnt" feeling you get when you have pushed beyond the limit so many times that you do not even know what the heck you are doing anymore. As Americans we are prone to going down in a metaphorical ball of flames rather often. We push ourselves to the brink and a lot of the time over the edge. Then we do as the shampoo bottle suggests and repeat the next day, and the next, and the next, and so forth.

To cleanse or to build...

That is a very important question!

Everywhere you look these days everyone has a hypothesis on whether to cleanse or build. These people keep trying to cram every person into some sort of mold. The person throws out that he or she is the foremost guru in so many years and they have shown the path of enlightenment to "x" amount of celebrities. The guru shouts, "You need to cleanse away the toxins that are depleting you!" We think, well maybe. The other guru shouts, "You must build up your body's reserves!" We think, quite possibly. So we get sucked into the infomercial at 3 am when our T – I – R – E – D bodies won't let us fall asleep. We cave in our disparity and order the guy's over-priced cure-all and wonder why it does nothing. Of course that's if we even open the package. Sometimes we let it sit on the shelf and forget it's even there.

To cleanse or to build? This is the question. This question can only be answered by each individual separately. Each person is different therefore each person needs to handle his/her plan on an individual basis. There are some basic guidelines to consider and possibly make the build or cleanse decision an easier one to make.

*Are you fatigued to the point of not being easily able to get going at the start of your day?

*Have you recently experienced a large amount of diarrhea or abdominal pain?

*Have you recently lost more than five pounds in a quick manner?

Answering yes to these three questions may indicate situations where harsh "cleansers " like herbal laxative formulas or kidney flushes or gall bladder cleanses may make you more run down than before you started. Look to more supportive or building products instead.

Seeking the advice of a person knowledgeable in the area of herbs and natural health is a good idea. If you have an on-going medical condition be
sure to discuss these choices with a medical practitioner.

I stand before you guilty of this practice. I have long since passed the safety zone of what my adrenals can handle, yet I push forward. I tend to run around like my hair is one fire, hence the cover image, with no end in sight. This happens to a vast number of "Type A" individuals. This book is an attempt to help those of you who have found yourself in a pile of ashes, needing to find a way to be reborn. And while there are men that fall in this category, there seems to be a larger number of women in this boat than guys. So while there are methods, hints, remedies, etcetera for everyone, you may find this read a bit geared more to the feminine. I apologize. I am female, though, so I happen to be better versed at how it works for us. But there is a plethora of information for all in the pages that follow.

RUSH and TIRED

"I am always tired."

"I never used to have to sleep so much!"

"No matter how much I sleep it's never enough."

"I just don't have time to be this darn tired!"

These are statements that I have heard from my clients in the last few years. They come to me seeking instant pep. They leave crushed because there is nothing I can give them that will energize them as quickly as they want. They are seeking a miracle in a pill and I don't have that. Unfortunately I do not think that exists and that type of thinking is dangerous. It can lead a person to dive headlong into any new thing that comes down the pike whether it is healthful for her or not.

Herbs, supplements and teas can enhance your body's ability to function but they cannot do the work alone. It takes time to rebuild a body. Think about how long it took to drive

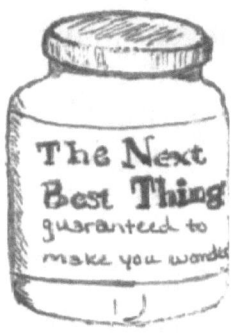

yourself into the hole you are in now. It didn't happen overnight. Therefore it will not be an overnight recovery either.

It seems that we get in a rut of RUSH and TIRED. We rush all over getting things done and in the process we end up making ourselves over-done. I like to think of the word rush as an acronym:

R eally

U nder –rested

S uper

H ectic

    This is the type of rush where you have one hour to clean your house for a meeting you committed to three months ago and had since forgotten about but are too ashamed to cancel due to having to admit you are not perfect. So you run around like a chicken with your head cut off slinging the babies' toys in a box and closet. You dig all the crap out from under your couch. *Oh my good gravy! What is that smell under your couch anyway?* You vacuum, throw together some pre-boxed munchies in a way that makes you feel like you went through countless hours of prepping by hand, and spray a ton of de-stinkifier spray around in hopes no one notices you haven't gotten to changing the fish tank filters in about six months or so. *Where's that spray stuff?* You forgot to allow time to shower, so now you just decide to plaster yourself with the spray, too. *What's that on the label? This stuff causes cancer in lab rats? No worries. You have no time for something that would consume so much of your time.* This is **R**eally **U**nder-rested **S**uper **H**ectic. This is the rush that will leave you T.I.R.E.D.

I think it is time to distinguish what kind of tired to which I refer. Every person on earth gets tired before they fall asleep, right? But what about the people that seems beyond the average tired? Here is the perfect acronym to remember exactly what kind of tired I wish to help people with:

T is for TOTALLY or TERRIBLY

I is for IRRITABLE and INSOMNIA

R is for RESTLESS or REALLY

E is for EXHAUSTED

D is for DEPRESSED and DYSFUNCTION

This acronym, a way to remember things like the nine planets or the ten cranial nerves, REALLY helps to illustrate the kind of rock bottom tired I'm talking about.

Anatomy of RUSH and TIRED

What bodily functions and mechanisms are we dealing with that leave us so run down? The body's chemical regulatory system is the eloquent symphony that keeps it all together. Hormones and glandular systems work in tandem with one another to keep the body moving. Let's take a look at this brilliant interaction starting from the top.

Your body's main control said for the hormonal system is in your head. The hypothalamus and pituitary gland kind of act like a set of tag-team air traffic controllers for the rest of the endocrine system. These two main players are responsible for which hormones and neurotransmitters are secreted and when. The hypothalamus tells the pituitary when to turn on or off and the pituitary then sends chemical messengers out to organ or gland specific targets.

These chemical messengers, called hormones, fit into the targets kind of like a key fits in a lock. Just like a square peg only fits in a square hole, these substances are what tell our organs how to behave. For example, the pituitary directs the adrenals to put out adrenal corticoid hormones. These hormones then work to regulate certain bodily functions like water balance, blood sugar levels, sex hormone levels, certain immune functions and more. Really, for how small the adrenal glands are, they are mighty little powerhouses that are vital to health regulation.

What's an adrenal gland? Oh my! You have been in a rush haven't you? These tiny glands are

The HPA Axis

The hypothalamus, pituitary and the adrenals communicate in something called the HPA axis. This network is kind of like a closed circuit communication network. The hypothalamus secretes hormones to the pituitary gland. The pituitary secretes hormones to the adrenals. The adrenals are then supposed to send messages back to the two superiors via a negative feedback loop.

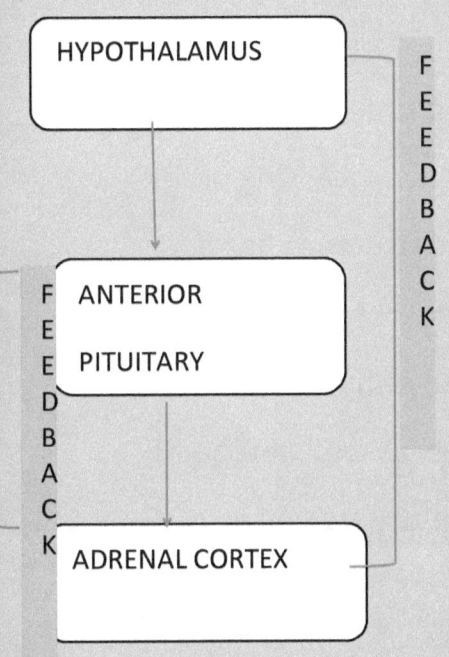

located on top of each kidney. Together they weigh about seven to ten grams. They work to secrete aldosterone, cortisol and androgens.

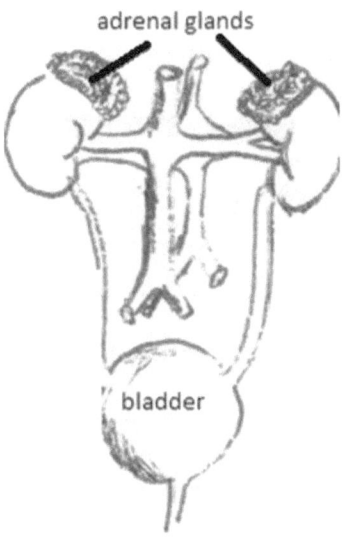

adrenal glands

bladder

In a normal stress response the body goes through some pretty heavy, lightening quick reactions. First the brain must perceive the happening as a stress. One person can be in a work environment where there is constant pressure to perform and her brain never perceives that as a threat. Another can be in the exact same environment and feel as if they are being attacked each and every day. During a stress response the hypothalamus secretes corticotrophin-releasing hormones. These are the messengers that tell the pituitary to kick it into high gear.

There is a structure in the brain called the amygdala that has to do with the processing of emotions. It is thought that this structure has a great deal to do with the entire stress response process, especially when fear and anxiety are involved. Other brain structures, as well, are being studied for their involvement in the triggering of stress responses. These structures like the hippocampus, Locus coeruleus, and the Raphe nucleus are now being shown to have a great deal to do with mood regulation and stress response functions.

The pituitary gland reacts to the emergency call by putting out adrenocorticotropic hormone. This is a very long term for a hormone that tells the adrenal glands to put out their hormones.

The adrenal hormones produced enable certain bodily reactions. Namely it puts out cortisol. Cortisol is the hormone that shunts sugar straight to the brain and muscles to aid in the ever popular fight-or-flight response. This is a great thing if you are confronted with by a hungry bear or by a mugger in a dark alley. This hormone allows you to do what you need to do to get yourself to a safe place.

When a person is constantly bombarded by stress, it is thought that this response fires over and over. The adrenal glands start to steadily release abnormally huge amounts of cortisol into the system. This leaves the person experiencing it tired and diminished. Then there is no reprieve. The response mechanisms fire over and over. The body is left craving sugar or other stimulants to function. Other side effects start to come to light as well, like cortisol's ability to suppress the immune system.

A "type A" personality person will be more prone to experiencing burnout than someone that is not. There are plenty of quizzes out there to find out if you may fall in this category. It is usually one of the things all undergrad psychology students have to do in at least one of their classes in college. Some good places to find quizzes to determine if you are a type A personality:

www.queendom.com

http://webspace.ship.edu/cgboer/jungiantypestest.html

http://pstypes.blogspot.com/2009/05/jung-test-type-evaluator.html

http://pstypes.blogspot.com/2009/03/free-jungian-type-tests.html

Some characteristics of a type A personality include:

Self-driven
Aggressive
Short tempered
Work-a-holic
Performance driven
Over-achiever
Irritated by loud, chaotic environments
Perfectionistic
Over-committing
Focused
Tightly clenched jaw
Pursed lips

This is not a definitive list, but gives you an idea as to what I am talking about.

"I just feel so fried..."

The over-activation of the stress response can result in a ton of symptoms. One of which is exhaustion. A more exact term would be over-exhaustion. This is more than pushing yourself to your "second wind." This is when you passed the fourth or fifth a few hours back.

To get a better understanding, let's look at the nervous system.

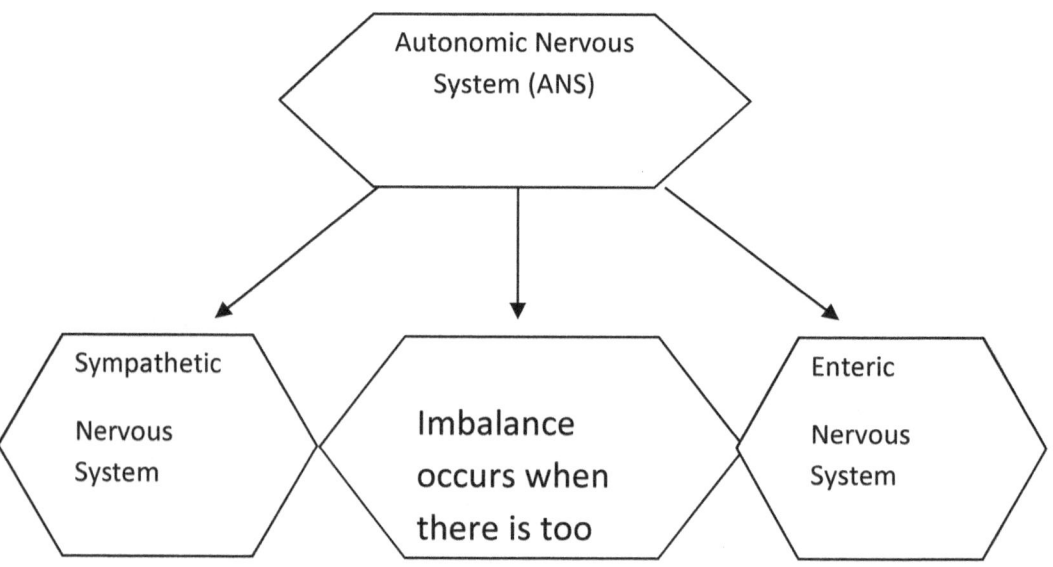

Autonomic Nervous System (ANS)

Sympathetic

Nervous System

Imbalance occurs when there is too

Enteric

Nervous System

The ANS is the network that controls involuntary and reflexive functions. It runs the internal organs like the heart, stomach and the intestines. It allows our heart rates to speed up or slow down, our blood vessels to dilate or contract, and certain muscles to contract or relax.

The previous chart illustrates the three main divisions of the ANS. These divisions need to be looked at when examining the lingering effects of constant adrenal stimulation. Stimulation of the adrenals in a stress response activates the Sympathetic Nervous System. This then causes the Parasympathetic nervous system to be repressed, at least momentarily. The next table illustrates the different actions that occur during the stimulation of either of the branches.

Structure	SNS stimulation	PNS stimulation
Iris/pupil	Pupil dilation	Pupil contraction
Salivary glands	Increased saliva	Decreased saliva
Mucosal membranes	Reduced mucus	Increased mucus
Heart	Increased rate and force	Decreased rate and force
Lungs	Bronchial muscles relax	Bronchial muscle contracts
Stomach	Peristalsis reduces	Peristalsis increases
Small intestine	Reduced motility	Increased motility
Large intestine	Reduced motility	Increased motility and

		secretions
Liver	Glycogen converts to glucose	
Kidney	Urine secretion reduces	Urine secretion increases
Adrenal medulla	Norepinephrine and epinephrine produced	
Bladder	Wall relaxed; sphincter closed	Wall contracts; sphincter relaxes

Source: http://faculty.washington.edu/chudler/auto.html, 12/5/2013

The ANS is always "on." It constantly is working in tandem with your somatic nervous system (the part of your nervous system that you "make" work. This is the voluntary control that you decide to make happen, like movement). It is said that the ANS is the part of your nervous system that is developed first in the womb.

Interestingly enough, in iridology it is taught that the ridge between the inner muscle body of the iris muscles and the ciliary body of muscles reflects the condition of the ANS. Whether or not you agree with the teachings of iridology, this is extremely interesting. What is even more interesting is that the areas representing the gut are contained inside this ridge. It is now known, through modern research, that the gut has its own nervous system. This gut-bound nervous system actually interacts with the ANS and plays a huge role in a person's behavior. I firmly believe that iridology is far beyond its time in being able to map a person's constitution and make-up. However, its weak point is that it is so varied, so diverse, that is impossible to scientifically prove any of it, at least at this time.

So why can't you sleep? People have a process going on called a Circadian Rhythm. In people that live typical daylight wakefulness routines, this rhythm means that cortisol (adrenal hormone) rises at about 8am and has its lowest points between 4pm and midnight. However, people that do not have this so-called "normal" schedule have issues.

These people are constantly exposed to extra stress. This extra stress raises adrenal stress response hormones (cortisol and adrenaline) at different times of the day than their bodies are programmed to experience. These hormones leave people hyper-vigilant or ready for a fight at a moment's notice. This leaves people on the edge of sleep and wakefulness. It leaves them in a difficult spot to relax into sleep like they possibly would if they did not have the complication of a second shift or night shift job.

Now, if the normal stresses that people deal with are added into this type of schedule and lack of sleep, then you end up with even more disbursements of adrenal hormones. This can bring about a compounding issue: blood sugar drops.

While cortisol can help to keep blood sugar levels at an even keel, fatigued adrenals (*woah...you mean they can get tired?* You bet they can) can put off cortisol in spurts. These spurts can work against a person trying to sleep, especially when the glycogen reserves in the liver are low. This drop in blood sugar then causes a person to wake up. They wake up and scavenge for food. How many people, including you, wake up in the middle of the night (between 1 am and 3 am) and go rooting around in the fridge for munchies? I have sleep eaters in my family. It causes me sixteen fits when I find plates, packages, and such by the side of their beds, etc.

You have all of this, add in a severe trauma. A death in the family, a sudden loss of a job, and/or a severe financial burden dropped on you, and you have the recipe for sleep destruction. Panic attacks, night terrors, and the like even add more burden to the adrenals.

Maybe you have inflicted this upon yourself? If one night of heavy drinking and no sleep don't kill you each week, then two or three or more won't either, right?

Forget ever sleeping. You find yourself grabbing over the counter medicines (chemicals) for sleep and then you feel so hung over from the meds that you go to caffeine and sugar laden wake-me-ups the next morning. *Don't tell me you have never tried a triple espresso mocha java latte. I know I have. I told you at the beginning, I have lived this.* This only leaves you burning quick energy and never touching glycogen stores, not do you restore those glycogen reserves.

And these aren't the only things, folks. The adrenals work in a partnership with the glands of your body. Remember those charts and diagrams earlier? All of the systems talk to each other. All of them act and react within a small universe of your body.

The next thing you know, you don't sleep without assistance. You can't even think past a shower without a cup – maybe a pot – of black coffee. Then you start noticing other things. You have scaly, flakes in your hair and on your cheeks. You have big, black bags under your eyes. You can't pee right nor do your bowels move without chemical assistance. You ache all over and feel way older than you really are. It doesn't take long to hit this point either. Once you hit this point, and think you have bounced back, it takes less and less time to hit the bottom again...and again...and again.

Resetting your sleep

Sleep is a huge issue. The CDC (Centers for Disease Control) has declared sleep deprivation a public health epidemic. Sleep deprivation has been associated with traffic accidents, on-the-job accidents, difficulty concentrating and more!

How do we get the adrenals to come back online, so to speak, to get sufficient sleep that makes us feel rested? How do we get that restful sleep that rejuvenates and restores us to the point where we wake up feeling refreshed and able to be productive during our day?

Let's start with the conventional points that the CDC and the regular medical community publicize regularly. Avoid caffeine, alcohol and nicotine, especially before bed. These things, in excess (*isn't America the home of excess*), can have negative effects on the adrenal gland's production of hormones. The small "boosts" you may feel from the excess production of adrenaline or other hormones can be easily pushed over the edge and burn out the adrenals ability to keep up. Alcohol especially can interfere with the glucose-glycogen cycles when used in excess.

Go to bed and wake up at the same time each night. Now, I laugh at this suggestion all the time. Really?!? In a world where more and more people are working multiple jobs or come from a home with both caregivers are working this becomes almost an impossible battle. I strive for this each day; however I am more than familiar with the impossibility of this very thing.

Eating a meal or a snack with high protein content can help steady the blood sugar levels to get through the night and can help prolong your sleep session.

Use supplements to increase the likelihood of achieving sleep. Supplements are not drugs. They are plants that contain certain chemical attributes that increase your body's natural ability to sleep.

Kava kava- Kava (*Piper methysticum*) is a Polynesian plant that has a long history of being used to produce a feeling of relaxation and has been used to promote sleep. This soporific or sedative quality is attributed to the kavalactones it contains.

It can be used in a variety of forms. The traditional use is as a drink that is made from the root. Traditionally it is used as a drink at various tribal-type celebrations in the Polynesian islands. It tends to produce a drunk-like result. Kava has been shown to reduce social anxiety better than a placebo in studies. It is suggested that people do not drive or operate heavy equipment when utilizing kava, similar to the precautionary directives given when imbibing alcoholic beverages.

It is commonly found in a capsule in the States. These capsules can be "standardized" for 30% to 90% kavalactones. It should be remembered that the traditional drinks, made in the way the Polynesians do, contains roughly 250 mg of kavalactones while these pills and capsules contain about 60 to 150 mg. So you should not expect the same feelings to come from uses the capsules as consuming the drink.

It should be mentioned that certain Kava supplements have been associated with liver damage. People should be sure that the Kava supplements they use come from the root, listed as rhizome on the label. The woody parts would be called the "aerial" parts on a label. Those aerial parts and the leaves are not the parts that are desired for relaxation. It is these aerial parts that can produce more liver toxicity than the root. As an added precaution people with compromised livers (cirrhosis, hepatitis, liver cancer, etc.) should not use Kava; nor should people on prescription medications that adversely affect the liver (certain statin drugs, blood thinners, etc.) use Kava. I consider Kava useful as a short-term use or intermittent use product that can give relief to random anxieties that interrupt sleep.

Hops- Hops (*Humulus lupulus*) is a wonderfully mild herb. It produces general relaxation. It is used in the brewing of beer and is a DISTANT relative of marijuana (*don't get any ideas. It is not the same thing*).

Hops has been through studies alone and with two other herbs I will go into shortly, Valerian and Passion Flower. While the studies were proclaimed inconclusive, I have found that it is quite beneficial for excitable children and elderly as a solo herb. It can aid in inducing the relaxation state necessary to achieve sleep.

Valerian- valerian root (*Valeriana officinalis*) is yet another herb that has been studied and the results have come back inclusive. I personally feel as if the results from all of these studies come back inconclusive because scientific personnel are trying to make one plant fit many people. I feel that if one plant was meant to fit the bill for all of the many peoples of the world, then we would not have all of these millions and billions of plants. It is impossible to say that one plant is going to be the one magic bullet that will fix all the ills of the world. Just the same, it is impossible to say that Valerian will fix all of the insomnia in the world. Different people react differently to different plants. Just like some people have reactions to a prescribed pharmaceutical that aids millions of people, some people have favorable responses to different plants than millions of other people. We, as people, need to stop trying to smash everyone into the same cookie cutter mold.

That being said, valerian root has been shown to produce sedative effects in animals, but as of the writing of this work, I was unable to find any document that has definitively found the chemical component responsible for this action. Darn! I guess that means the pharmaceutical industry cannot isolate that one component and synthetically produce it.

Valerian has an unmistakable odor that kind of resembles teenaged boy gym bag. Remember, it is a swamp plant. As swamps are not exactly odorifically beautiful, neither is valerian. As an herbalist, I have been trained to look for this smell. If you buy a valerian supplement that does not smell like dirty sweaty socks, you have been sold a bogus supplement. As a side note, opening the capsules of valerian in hot water and making a tea from the dried herb, rids it of the characteristic odor and makes it slightly more palatable.

Passion flower- passion flower (*Passiflora incarnata)* has been used for some time to reduce anxiety and aid for those experiencing mild insomnia. While the National Institutes for Health say the results for passion flower's effectiveness are inconclusive, it also then contradicts itself by saying the chemical components of passion flower do that very thing. Once again, a case of a scientific body trying to shove everyone into the same cookie cutter mold rears its head.

That being said, scientists believe that passion flower may increase the production of a neurotransmitter called GABA. GABA (gamma aminobutyric acid) actually stops and/or slows down some of the activity of some brain cells thereby inducing relaxation.

Passion flower is often used in combination with other herbs. One of my absolutely favorite blends combines this plant, used since before the Spanish conquistadors came to the New World, with valerian and hops. Another wonderful blend uses those three with a mix of essential minerals and vitamins for the adrenal glands.

Increasing energy & stamina

One thing that seems to go hand in hand with adrenal exhaustion is low energy and stamina. If you used to be able to run a mile, but now you just can't hack it, you could benefit from a look at your adrenals. Even on a more basic level, if you used to be able to pull an over-nighter at work and get up and go the next day, but now it plows you under for the next 48 hours, you really need to look at your adrenals.

You didn't end up tired and weak by just one instance of burning the candle at both ends. I know I didn't. I really did not comprehend what was going on with me until I was at a meeting and a check list was presented to adequately measure

the life stressors that people are exposed to.

That check list is below and can be found at

http://www.roadtowellbeing.ca/questionnaires/life-stressors.html

Life Event	Points
Death of spouse	100
Son or daughter leaving home	29
Divorce	73
Trouble with in-laws	29
Marital separation	65
Outstanding personal achievement	28
Jail term	63
Spouse begins or ceases working	26
Death of close family member	63
Starting or finishing school	26
Personal injury or illness	53
Change in living conditions	25
Marriage	50
Revision of personal habits	24
Fired from job	47
Trouble with boss	23
Marital reconciliation	45
Change in work hours, conditions	20
Retirement	45
Change in residence	20
Change in family member's health	44
Change in schools	20
Pregnancy	40
Change in recreational habits	19
Sexual difficulties	39
Change in church activities	19

Addition to family	39
Change in social activities	18
Business readjustment	39
Mortgage or loan under $10, 000	17
Change in financial status	38
Change in sleeping habits	15
Death of close friend	37
Change in number of family gatherings	15
Career change	36
Change in eating habits	15
Change in # of marital arguments	35
Vacation	13
Mortgage or loan over $10,000	31
Christmas season	12
Foreclosure of mortgage or loan	30
Minor violation of the law	11
Change in work responsibilities	29

For each one of these life events, add the points assigned to it. I had no idea just how far in I really was until I added all of my points and ended up with 724. The guy teaching the meeting stopped the class and gave me three free bottles of supplements for my adrenals.

The point is we have real problems every single day. It is how we react to these and the accumulative effects of these things and events that determine our adrenal health. Each and every event can take a chunk of your energy away until you end up like me, a ball of sick and tired mush. I did it to myself in high school and did not realize the impact until a car accident put me over the edge. That was the event that sent me searching for herbal alternatives (well...my doctor told my mother to find another way because he refused to put me on SSRI's). In my adult life, it was difficult to not slip back into that Type-A behavior and wound up there once again. I can't be the only person with a bit of a Wonder Woman complex.

How do we get that energy back? First of all, sleep deprivation must be addressed (see previous section). While the CDC says the average amount of sleep for adults is eight hours (seven to nine to be exact), those with a history of burnt adrenals will probably require more each day and may even require brief periods of "sleep banking."

Sleep banking is what I call the extreme sleep periods of more than 12 hours when the body just needs to rejuvenate. If these happen frequently, other issues must be addressed, including disease or clinical depression and require a visit to a licensed medical professional. However, once in a while, my body just shuts down and needs to refill the bank.

Circadian Rhythm

It may be helpful here to take a quick look at a "normal" circadian rhythm. This is the term used to refer to the "biological clock" that governs the body's processes, like sleep. Below is a chart that illustrates a "normal" circadian rhythm.

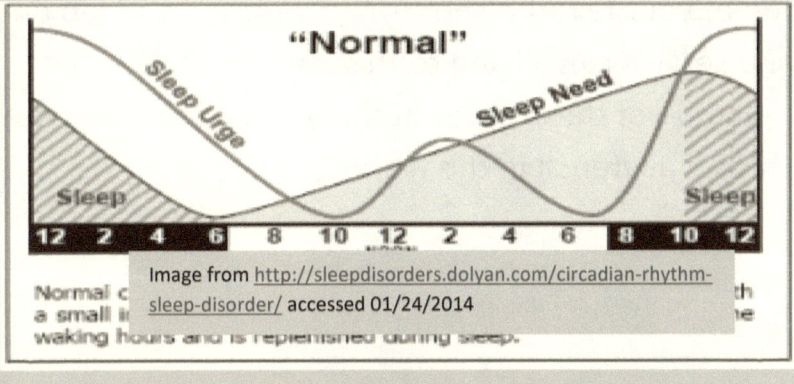

Image from http://sleepdisorders.dolyan.com/circadian-rhythm-sleep-disorder/ accessed 01/24/2014

The problem comes when the HPA that we went over earlier is on chronic over-drive. This is when the levels of ACTH (Adrenocorticotropic hormone) and cortisol are elevated for prolonged periods of time. These prolonged periods are longer than what is seen in the "normal" person that would display a "normal" circadian rhythm (see previous illustration).

Several studies cite the correlation between the over stimulation of the central nervous system and the disturbance of the circadian rhythm. What they disagree on is whether the lack of sleep made the over-stimulation or the over-stimulation made the lack of sleep. I say it is caused by both. Life is a two-way street after all. There is no hard and fast rule, that I am aware of, that states this is not possible. All of those perceived threats can add up. All of those late nights cramming for exams, baking your kids' brownies, working a night shift with no sleep the next day, and/or getting in one more episode of your favorite show on your favorite video on demand service can all add to this imbalance. IT is the accumulation of these types of things on a regular basis that throws a wrench in the works.

Many sources suggest the elimination of caffeine to boost energy. I know from experience that just dropping this substance can produce terrible symptoms including headaches, nausea, tremors, and more exhaustion. I find it better to reduce caffeine gradually. Are you a coffee drinker? Try switching to yerba mate. It has a coffee like taste, some caffeine, and more antioxidants than plain coffee. Another option is switch to a blend of roasted chicory and dandelion root. Many people swear that this blend is identical in taste to coffee and is definitely better for you.

Are you a cola drinker? Try tea or tea blends. Colas, when consumed on a regular basis, can be just as addictive as any other substance. The fizzy taste and the high quantities of sugar (or artificial sweeteners) can cause severe withdraw symptoms. Homemade soda machines are affordable now and it is plausible to make your own soda containing stevia, or stevia derived sweeteners, which have less glycemic impact. Be sure to check your non-cola sodas for caffeine, too. Many root beers and orange sodas have added caffeine to increase the "bite" of the drink. However, the acids contained in carbonated sodas can eat away the enamel of your teeth. So it is a great idea to never start consuming them on a regular basis in the first place.

Green tea has become a relatively easy beverage to find. It is available in many blends and as an addition to many other drinks. While green tea has some caffeine in it, the level is less than coffee and less than that in colas. It contains something called EGCG which has been shown to be of benefit in weight loss, and many antioxidant polyphenols.

Theanine is a component of green tea that has been shown in recent studies to decrease the effects of stress on cognitive functioning. Stressed lab rats that were fed theanine showed better cognitive functioning than those that were not fed the green tea component. What more reasons are needed to add this beverage to your routine?

Light therapy has shown some promise in helping people get back on the track to proper rest and energy cycles. Several sources indicate the use of full spectrum lights (special bulbs that emit the same frequencies of light as the sun) for this type of thing. The light, and the special spectrum emitted, makes the body produce melatonin. Melatonin is the body's own sleep producing hormone. While it is possible to take melatonin as a supplement in the US and as a prescription medication in some other countries, I prefer to stay away from it if possible. There have been some studies indicating that long-term or regular use of it may interfere with the body's ability to produce its own melatonin.

If you think about it, this is a very feasible idea. People do not spend as much time outside as they did just 20 years ago. We cloister ourselves indoors, staring at a computer screen (not a full spectrum light by any means) for countless hours with limited sunlight exposure and little to no physical activity and wonder why we can't sleep.

This brings me to the topic of exercise. Exercise has been shown to increase energy and vitality. The trick is to be consistent. Starting slowly and building up to more vigorous exercise does help the body learn to secrete various endorphins (feel good hormones) and regulates adrenal secretions. On a side note: no one cares if you look silly at the gym or how much you weigh while you are there. You are there to exercise, then quit worrying about what other people think and get your buns moving.

Crabby Pants

I don't know about you, but when I am in burn out mode I am a real bitch. People that are adrenal fatigued are crabby. They don't want to be bothered. These people don't want to be coerced, enticed nor do they want to be annoyed. They are experiencing the "I" from our TIRED model.

This could be due to the adrenals' effect on the blood sugar levels as well as the lack of quality sleep. The fatigued adrenal glands put out cortisol and adrenaline in spurts. This causes abnormal highs and lows that can make it difficult to stay asleep, as discussed previously.

Research has found that cortisol and progesterone (the "feel-good" pregnancy related hormone) compete for receptor sites in the brain.

Hormones fit into receptor sites kind of like a key fits in a lock. Sometimes, they almost function like the old fashioned locks and keys. There may be a best fitting key, but a skeleton key can fit every lock in the house and fit when the others cannot be found. When your body has an excess of cortisol, it will grab it up instead of progesterone.

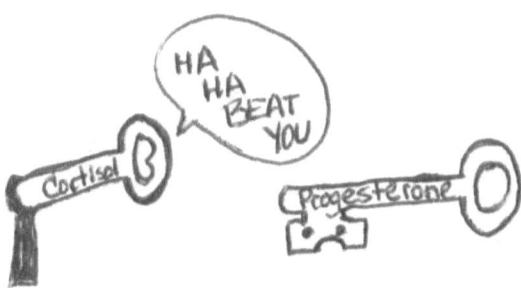

Cortisol does not balance the other hormones in the body and you could be left feeling symptoms that have been described as "estrogen dominance."

According to Dr. Christine Northrup, the symptoms of estrogen dominance are:

- Decreased sex drive
- Irregular or otherwise abnormal menstrual periods
- Bloating
- Breast swelling and tenderness
- Fibrocystic breasts
- Headaches
- Mood swings (irritability, depression)
- Weight and/or fat gain (especially abdomen and hips)
- Cold hands and feet (possibly thyroid dysfunction)
- Hair loss
- Thyroid dysfunction
- Sluggish metabolism
- Foggy thinking, memory loss
- Fatigue

- Trouble sleeping/insomnia

- PMS
(list from
http://www.drnorthrup.com/womenshealth/healthcenter/topic_details.php?topic_id=1
18, accessed 2/5/2014)

Experiencing these symptoms while leading up to menopause should be a flare shot into the night sky for doctors, but sometimes they miss it. They sound a lot like the symptoms of adrenal fatigue, don't they? There are actually studies out there that have found activity (physical and mental) and stress levels through perimenopause to be one determining factor of the severity of menopausal symptoms like hot flashes, irritability, and brain fog. One such study, which I found in a past issue of the Journal of Women's Health, actually cites decreased adrenal function as a possible reason for menopausal discomfort.

There are herbs to aid you in the quest to bring you back to your same old self.

Some experts point to adrenal function decreases as the underlying cause of PMS. The symptoms of PMS eerily sound like those listed above for estrogen dominance, don't they?

Wild Yam (*Dioscorea villosa*) has been historically used to balance these levels. Progesterone creams made from diosgenin have been quite popular for use in balancing these symptoms. Be sure to find a cream that meets the recommendations of Dr. John Lee, a foremost researcher on the topic of estrogen dominance. Pro-G-Yam cream is just one that supplies these suggested ingredients.

Singing the fatigued blues...

Maybe these remedies can help.

St. John's Wort (*Hypericum perforatum*) has received a mixed-bag of reviews. Lauded as a remedy for depression in the 1990's, it has been shown to be as effective as selective-serotonin reuptake inhibitors (SSRI's) and certain tricyclic antidepressants for mild to moderate depression. A word of caution here: medical professionals suggest you do not mix St. John's Wort with these medications. You really should consult your mental health physician and your pharmacist if you are using prescribed medications for depression or any mental illness before you mix in herbs like St. John's Wort.

Should you consider switching to herbs instead of your prescription, please be aware that I do not condone this action unless you discuss it with your doctor that prescribed the medication (or the one you are currently seeing for that condition) and he/she consents and monitors your transition.

For those that are not on medications, then give this herb a try. It does so much more than just brighten your mood. Also known as Klammath Weed, it has been historically used to treat burns. Klammath Weed oil is made by soaking the yellow flowers in an oil like olive oil. It then turns a red color. It should be noted that this remedy has not be medically tested, but the plant has shown to have activity against gram-positive bacteria in lab settings.

I have used the alcohol based extract in a transdermal, or poultice, delivery. As a teenager, I suffered from many periods of "stomach flu." These left me with gut wrenching cramps and diarrhea. It was suggested by one of the local herbalists, with which I was working, to put the extract in my belly button and let it "soak in." I was pretty skeptical. At that point I did not believe that anything natural would be of any benefit unless ingested. I am happy to report that this did take the edge off of the gripping pains and helped me get back on my feet.

It relaxes my gut. This is great as I, as well as many people recovering from adrenal burn-out and fatigue, seem to suffer from irritable bowel or other inflammatory conditions of the alimentary canal.

There is a huge list of medications with which to not use this herb. Please check it out with your pharmacist to be sure you are not at risk.

Damiana (*Turnera diffusa*) is another herb I find beneficial. It helps to "brighten" the mood. In fact, my clients that have used it have reported feeling almost giddy. While this native Mexican shrub has been vilified by some, it has been traditionally used as an aphrodisiac and generally tonic to make people happy. There are few studies showing any evidence one way or the other for this herb. It is suggested to avoid this herb if you are diabetic or on medication to treat medically diagnosed blood sugar disorders.

I have read that Damiana may be a controlled substance in some states in the U.S. I am not aware of this being an issue, and certainly do not know why it would be. I have never heard of any instances of substance abuse-like situations, but be aware of what your local laws state. I do not suggest anyone break a law.

My favorite way to use Damiana is via decoction, or making it into a tea. While capsules are an extremely convenient way to get herbs into your system, using this one as a tea decreases absorption time. And who doesn't need to take a step back with a nice cup of tea from time to time?

Anxious days and nights

Remember that mugger that is nowhere to be found? Those types of feelings induce plenty of anxiety. The feeling that you are "Waiting for the other shoe to fall" or that there will be another impending disaster can stress a person out, which in turn elevates cortisol levels.

Anxiety can also be the flip side of the depression coin. According to the Anxiety and Depression Society of America, anxiety is the most common mental illness in the United States. They put the number effected at 40 million adults aged 18 and up. That's about 18% of the population. That's a lot of anxious people. Half of those diagnosed with anxiety are also diagnosed with depression.

It is almost as if anxiety leads to depression and visa versa. It's a cyclical mental disorder that encompasses a ton of factors including genetics, environment and more.

Mental disorders result in many trips to medical doctors. The soaring costs and side-effect reports of pharmaceutical psycho-active medications have prompted many to look for nutritional support for these types of symptoms.

It is difficult to find research supporting the use of herbs and vitamin and mineral supplements to aid in these instances. However, I did find one that not only recommended two of the herbs mentioned earlier, Passion Flower and Kava, but it also mentioned the use of two wonderful amino acids for reducing anxiety. L-lysine and L-arginine have been used by some with successful results. A placebo controlled, double blind study found on Pubmed.gov points out that these two amino acids may very well be effective for healthy adults to use in order to combat high levels of mental anxiety. They measured the salivary cortisol of the participants and found that those using these supplements during times of increased mental stress and anxiety had lower cortisol levels. That means the adrenal glands were better able to cope with the stresses.

Magnesium has also been mentioned by some to help with feelings of anxiety. Magnesium has been shown to act as an inhibitor to prevent certain other elements to bind to receptors and cause excited responses, like anxiety. Magnesium has been shown to reduce blood pressure and other anxiety co-symptoms. Most American diets fall short in Magnesium levels and therefor set up in an already deficient state, afflicting us with an Achilles'' heel when it comes to dealing with stress and anxiety. Most sources suggest a dose of about 400 mg each day.

B vitamins are my favorite class of vitamins. There are so many ways lose these vital nutrients. B vitamins are water soluble. This means your body can only hold on to so much at one time. The excess is excreted via urine, sweat and feces.

How do we avoid this loss of B's? Constant ingestion is the only way. They are vital to so many bodily functions that many books have been written and devoted solely to B vitamins. The Standard American Diet (SAD) is devoid of many B vitamins and contains so many refined foods and starches that many of the B's we do take in are lost just trying to get the body balanced.

B vitamins feed your adrenals. Vitamin B5 (Pantothenic Acid) is turned in to a substance that is vital for the transformation of glucose into energy. Most sources suggest starting at 1500 mg per day for a normal adult.

Niacin is an essential nutrient in the synthesis of adrenal hormones used in adrenal responses. It makes the reactions happen in some of the crucial steps. Some sources suggest 25 to 50 mg per day to ensure you get enough niacin each day. However, niacin can dilate the blood vessels and cause a flushing reaction, not unlike a menopausal hot flash. If this would happen to occur, seek out niacinmide. This form of the crucial B vitamin does not cause the hot flushing reaction and is of extreme benefit.

B6 is a rather popular B vitamin. I first encountered use of it in my own life while pregnant with my oldest son. It has the ability to thwart water retention. Since it has diuretic actions it is often used by those individuals looking to rid him or her of joint swelling.

One indicator for whether or not you might need vitamin B6 is if you remember your dreams.

If you cannot, it is suggested you take about 50-100 mg of this vital B.

Don't forget B Complex. While each of these three B vitamins is in B Complex, the entire package is necessary to get the single ones to do their job. It's kind of like the Complex is the bus that gets the motor club to the broken down car. This where the individual specialist get out of the bus and fix your vehicle. If B Complex is the bus, Pantothenic Acid, niacin and B6 are the specialists.

Vitamin C is another water soluble vitamin that aids the adrenals in producing the hormones needed to keep up with stress and anxiety responses. It should be consumed throughout the day as opposed to one giant burst. You will only soak up so much at one time with the rest going, literally, down the toilet. I once heard that the dried adrenal gland is made up of a huge amount of vitamin C. I am not sure of the truth of this, but it has helped me remember the importance of feeding vitamin C to the adrenals.

There is a blend I like to use that works better than anything else I have ever found and includes all of these vitamins, minerals and my three favorite herbs, valerian, passion flower and hops. Nutri-Calm is that supplement. This supplement takes the speed bumps out of the day of the anxiety prone and lifts, ever-so-slightly, the spirits of the depressed. There are few people, in my opinion, that do not benefit from Nutri-Calm.

Heart-stress connection

Although Western or modern medicine does not acknowledge a lot of what Traditional Chinese Medicine has to offer, there is something to be said about the connection between stress and the function of the circulatory system. More specifically, this connection involves the adrenals and the heart.

Ever notice how stress affects everyone differently? In some individuals, these continuous stresses can aggravate the blood pressure. You see, in Traditional Chinese Medicine (TCM) the heart houses the mind. By "mind" I am talking about the *thinking* mind, not the *doing* mind.

It is no coincidence, then, that there exists a standard recipe of herbs in TCM that helps with "heart stress." This combination, called yang xin (nurture heart), contains schizandra fruit, biota seed, cistanche stem, cuscuta seed, lycium fruit, ophiopogon root tuber, succinum amber, tang-kuei root, acorus rhizome, astragalus root, dioscorea rhizome, hoelen sclerotium, lotus seed, ginseng root, polygala root, polygonatum rhizome, jujuba seed and rehmannia root tuber.

This is one of my most used remedies. A sure signal an individual could benefit from this combination is found using tongue analysis (sometimes referred to as tongue diagnosis).

In this analysis method, the tongue is examined to determine a most current state of the body. The area of the very tip of the tongue corresponds to the mind, which in TCM is the heart. If this tip is very red in contrast to the rest of the tongue, I consider suggesting yang xin as a remedy. If the tongue seems to uncontrollably quiver or shake, then I certainly urge the client to use the formula. If the client says he or she suffers from high blood pressure, I put the remedy in his or her hand and they usually try it with much success.

A word about

TCM (Traditional Chinese Medicine)

TCM is an invaluable tool for mankind. This system of healing has existed thousands of years. We are just now finding scientific support for the remedies used in this ancient system.

In TCM, every organ and every system is thought to interact and interplay with each other by balancing Chi (energy). Both positive and negative chi is present at all times. This ying and yang represents the ebb and flow of vitality present in all bodily components.

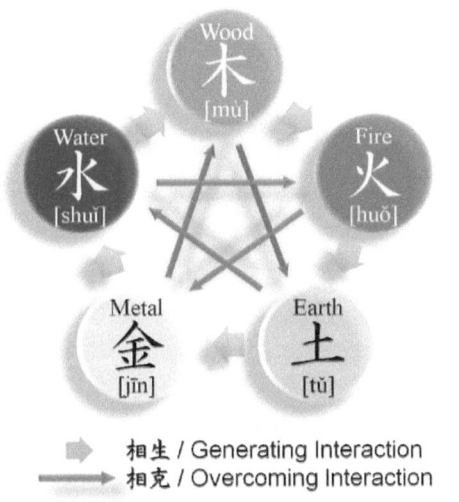

5 elements chart from http://en.wikipedia.org/wiki/File:Wu_Xing.png . 03/21/2014

"Bio-identical" hormones

Hormones are big news as of late. Several pharmacies now compound hormone "replacement" medications for women. While this can be of benefit, one should use these medications with just as caution as any other prescription based hormonal treatment.

Often these synthetic hormones are touted as "bio-identical" hormones. There is nothing 100% identical about them. "bio-similar" would be a name for them. I personally view these, sometimes animal derived, hormones as a half-step between herbal and pharmaceutical.

I like to try all natural as much as possible. If that does not work, then I would most definitely graduate to the "bio-similar" hormones next. Please be aware that these hormones do still require a licensed medical doctor's prescription and can only be obtained from compounding pharmacies.

The light at the end of the tunnel

I know the things in this short book seem like a lot to incorporate into your life. There is a light at the end of this tunnel you feel like you have been stuck in, though. There is relief and you can regain your balance. Remember, it did not take just one single instance of stress to put your adrenals over the edge. Rather, it was repeated abuses and the constant pushing of limits that landed you in the exhaustion phase in which you now find yourself.

Likewise, it will take some time to get you built back up. Working to re-establish restorative sleep, knowing your limitations and boundaries, learning to say no, and other self-preservation methods can help you rebuild and find your vitality.

You may not be able to scale a tall mountain in a single jaunt, but many small goes at it may produce a great accomplishment, and leave you better able to tell the tale after.

SOURCES:

http://faculty.washington.edu/chudler/auto.html, 12/5/2013

www.adrenalfatiguefocus.org, 12/6/2013

http://www.adrenalfatigue.org/sleep-disruption, 01/01/2014

http://www.ncbi.nlm.nih.gov/pubmed/23458739 , 02/13/2014

http://www.cdc.gov/features/dssleep/ 01/01/2014

Pittler MH, Ernst E (2003). "Kava extract for treating anxiety". In Pittler, Max H. *Cochrane database of systematic reviews (Online)* (1): CD003383. doi:10.1002/14651858.CD003383. PMID 12535473.

http://www.healthline.com/natstandardcontent/hops 01/01/2014

http://ods.od.nih.gov/factsheets/Valerian-HealthProfessional/ 01/01/2014

http://www.nlm.nih.gov/medlineplus/druginfo/natural/871.html 01/01/2014

http://www.roadtowellbeing.ca/questionnaires/life-stressors.html 01/01/2014

http://www.roadtowellbeing.ca/questionnaires/life-stressors.html 01/04/2014

http://my.clevelandclinic.org/neurological_institute/sleep-disorders-center/disorders-conditions/hic-circadian-rhythm-disorders.aspx 01/26/2014

http://my.clevelandclinic.org/neurological_institute/sleep-disorders-center/disorders-conditions/hic-circadian-rhythm-disorders.aspx 01/26/2014

http://www.webmd.com/sleep-disorders/guide/circadian-rhythm-disorders-cause 01/26/2014

http://www.aasmnet.org/resources/factsheets/crsd.pdf 01/26/2014

Buckley TM, Schatzberg AF. On the interactions of the hypothalamic-pituitary-adrenal (HPA) axis and sleep: normal HPA axis activity and circadian rhythm, exemplary sleep disorders. J Clin Endocrinol Metab. 2005 May;90(5):3106-14. Epub 2005 Feb 22.

Vgontzas AN, Bixler EO, Lin HM, Prolo P, Mastorakos G, Vela-Bueno A, Kales A, Chrousos GP. Chronic insomnia is associated with nyctohemeral activation of the hypothalamic-pituitary-adrenal axis: clinical implications. J Clin Endocrinol Metab. 2001 Aug;86(8):3787-94.

http://naturopathconnect.com/articles/circadian-rhythm-disorder-symptoms/ 01/26/2014

http://stanfordhospital.org/clinicsmedServices/clinics/sleep/treatment_options/bright-light-therapy.html 01/26/2014

http://www.mayoclinic.org/tests-procedures/light-therapy/basics/definition/prc-20009617 01/26/2014

http://yoursleep.aasmnet.org/Treatment.aspx?id=4 01/26/2014

http://www.johnleemd.com/store/pms_stress.html 02/05/2014

http://www.drnorthrup.com/womenshealth/healthcenter/topic_details.php?topic_id=118 02/05/2014 http://www.mayoclinic.org/drugs-supplements/st-johns-wort/background/hrb-20060053 02/05/2014

http://www.drugs.com/mtm/damiana.html 02/05/2014

Sarasohn, Lisa, The Woman's Belly Book. New World Library, Novato, Caslifornia. 2006

http://www.adaa.org/about-adaa/press-room/facts-statistics 02/05/2014

Brian W. Whitcomb, Maura K. Whiteman, Patricia Langenberg, Jodi A. Flaws, and William A. Romani. Journal of Women's Health. January/February 2007, 16(1): 124-133. doi:10.1089/jwh.2006.0046.

Lakhan, Shaheen E, Karen F Vieira. Nutritional and herbal supplements for anxiety and anxiety-related disorders: systematic review. Lakhan and Vieira Nutrition Journal 2010, 9:42 http://www.nutritionj.com/content/9/1/42

http://www.ncbi.nlm.nih.gov/pubmed/17510493 02/13/2014

http://www.psychologytoday.com/blog/evolutionary-psychiatry/201106/magnesium-and-the-brain-the-original-chill-pill 02/13/2014

http://www.ncbi.nlm.nih.gov/pubmed/23603926 02/13/2014

http://altmedicine.about.com/cs/anxietydepression/a/EmotionsTCM.htm 03/21/14

Resources:

Let's face it, sometimes finding this stuff isn't easy. Where are the best places to find the things listed in this little book? The first place I would start is my local health food store. If you have no luck there, check out the following information. I want to make sure you get a hold of all the things you seek.

Herbal Beverage- a natural coffee replacement made from a roasted chicory blend. Can be found at herbchick.mynsp.com, stock number 1600-1.

Nutri-Calm- a supplement containing vitamin C, thiamin (B1), riboflavin (B2), niacin, B6, folic acid, B12, biotin and pantothenic acid, plus schizandra fruit, choline, inositol, bee pollen, PABA, lemon bioflavonoids, valerian root extract, passionflower flowers extract and hops flowers extract. Can be found at herbchick.mynsp.com, stock number 1617-3.

Kava Kava- can be found at herbchick.mynsp.com, stock number 405-9

Pro-G-Yam Cream- can be found at herbchick.mynsp.com, stock number 4948-0

Valerian root -can be found at herbchick.mynsp.com, stock number 720-0

Passion Flower- can be found at herbchick.mynsp.com, stock number 500-3

Hops- can be found at herbchick.mynsp.com, stock number 380-9

St. John's Wort- can be found at herbchick.mynsp.com, stock number 655-3

St. John's Wort Kudzu- can be found at herbchick.mynsp.com, stock number 975-4

Damiana- can be found at herbchick.mynsp.com, stock number 240-9

Heart stress formula yang xin- can be found at herbchick.mynsp.com, stock number 1884-7

Pubmed.gov -This government supported website hosts information on studies investigating the uses of various natural and alternative health avenues. Subscription and access to the information is free. Sign up at http://www.pubmed.gov.

NCCAM -This is the National Center for Complementary and Alternative Medicine. This is the branch of the National Institute of Health that investigates various natural, alternative and complimentary health modalities. It is funded by the United States Government and is the agency responsible for the pubmed.gov postings.

DSHEA-
The Dietary Supplement Health and Education act of 1994. This act clearly sets the FDA as the regulatory body over both finished dietary supplement products and dietary ingredients. While the FDA regulates dietary supplements under a different set of regulations than those covering "conventional" foods and drug products, the act sets these guidelines, among others:

"Manufacturers and distributors of dietary supplements and dietary ingredients are prohibited from marketing products that are adulterated or misbranded. That means that these firms are responsible for evaluating the safety and labeling of their products before marketing to ensure that they meet all the requirements of DSHEA and FDA regulations.

FDA is responsible for taking action against any adulterated or misbranded dietary supplement product after it reaches market." (Quote taken directly from http://www.fda.gov/Food/Dietarysupplements/default.htm, accessed 03/21/2014)

www.ingramcontent.com/pod-product-compliance
Lightning Source LLC
Chambersburg PA
CBHW020350290526
45785CB00005B/2218